Understanding Lean And Green Diet

The Complete Guide To Fueling Hacks & Lean And Green Recipes To Help You Keep Healthy And Lose Weight By Harnessing The Power Of Lean And Green Meals

Natalie Allen

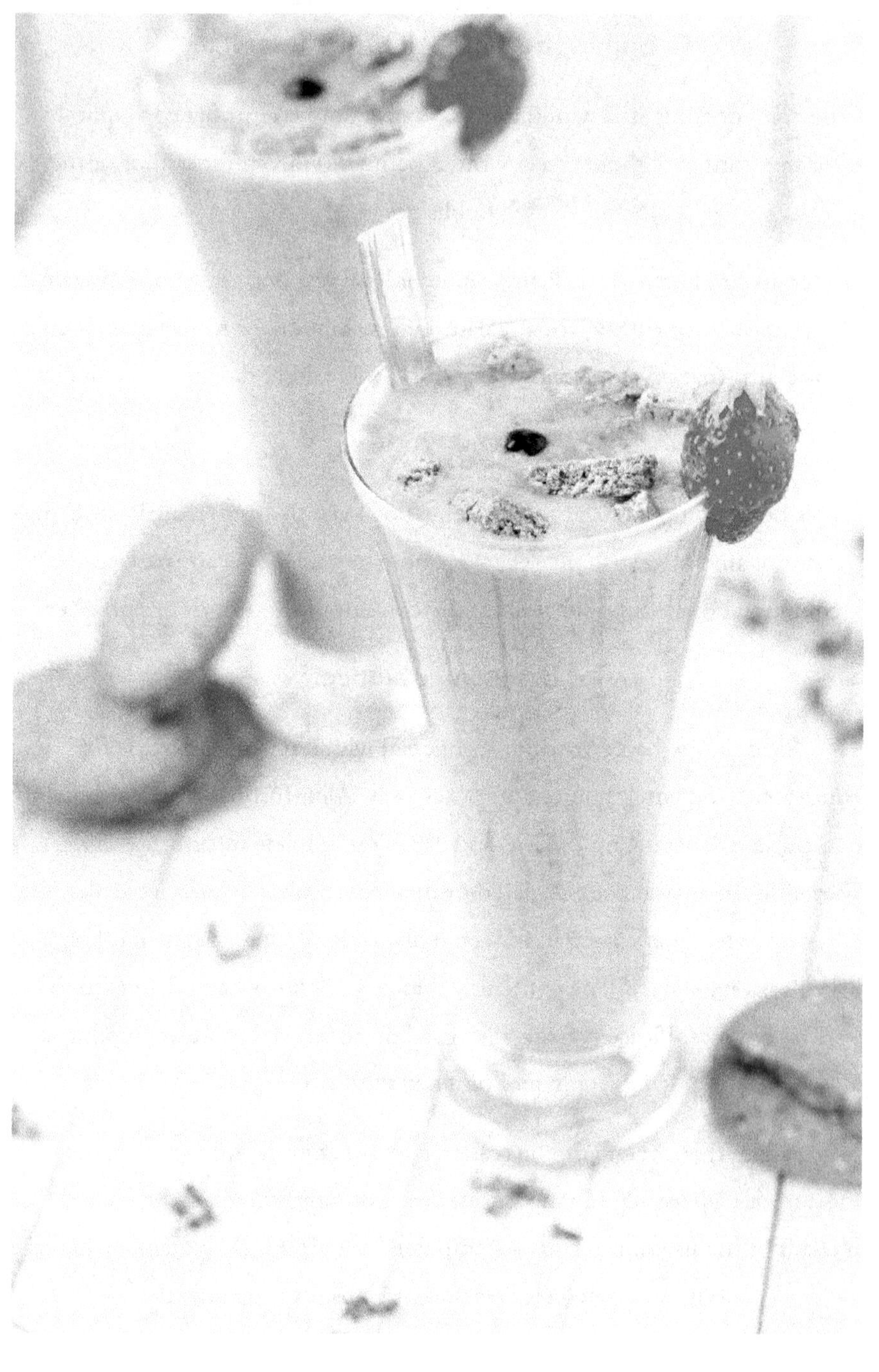

TABLE OF CONTENTS

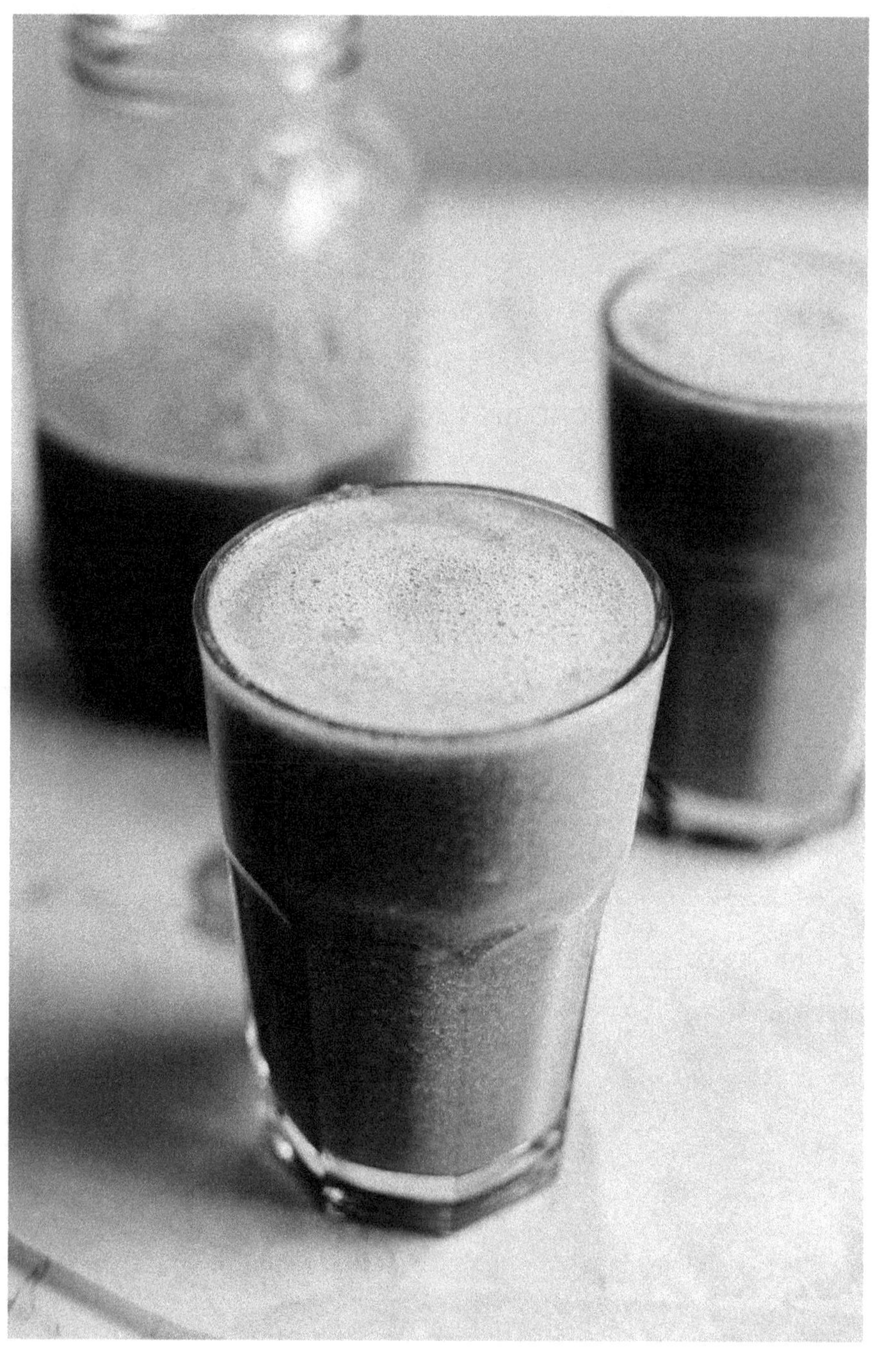

Introduction

One way is by changing your diet and cooking in a smarter way. Lean and Green Cookbook provides recipes for delicious, healthy food with reduced environmental impact. Get ready to cook up a storm that's good for the environment!

This article was written because there are so many people who want tips and tricks on how to stay lean while reducing their environmental impact. It does not matter if you are a novice or a pro chef; this book will educate and inspire a way to make the best out of the foods you eat. Eat healthy with dietary guidelines in mind. s

The cookbook is full of a little bit of everything from main dishes to light breakfasts. From protein-packed animal and seafood recipes to balanced and delicious vegetarian and vegan dishes. So, get ready for a feast on the go! You'll be amazed just how tasty healthy can be in a nutshell.

Lean and Green is perfect for people who want to cook healthy food without a lot of hassle or spending a lot of time in the kitchen. It includes easy recipes that take 30 minutes or less to make, making it ideal for busy people with hectic schedules. In addition, the book is also loaded with nutritional information about every recipe, including calories, fat, carbohydrates, and protein content.

Vegetarian Delicacies: Everything you need to know about vegetarian cuisine. These dishes include Mexican, Italian, Chinese, Indian, Thai, Greek, French, Japanese, and Taiwanese. The recipes are based on traditional food from these countries that are healthy without being bland or boring. These recipes are also vegan and gluten-free.

Everything you need to know about vegetarian cuisine. These dishes include Mexican, Italian, Chinese, Indian, Thai, Greek, French, Japanese and Taiwanese. The recipes are based on traditional food from these countries that are healthy without being bland or boring. These recipes are also vegan and gluten-free. Heartiest Dishes: These dishes are full of protein and carbohydrates as well as vitamins and minerals. The meals are hearty but leave you feeling full so you don't need to eat constantly. They feature a variety of meats, beans and vegetables. These dishes make great entrees or side dishes.

These dishes are full of protein and carbohydrates as well as vitamins and minerals. The meals are hearty but leave you feeling full so you don't need to eat constantly. They feature a variety of meats, beans and vegetables. These dishes make great entrees or side dishes. Energy Boosts: These dishes are tasty and nutritious but also relatively low in calories. They will provide the boost you need to recover from a hard workout or day at work.

Most people don't have time to cook healthy food, but that doesn't mean it's out of the question. On the contrary, people should always be trying to incorporate healthy eating into their lives. There are many ways for you to do this, such as making changes to your diet or stocking your pantry with nutritious ingredients. This will help you better control your diabetes and overall health.

21 Days Meal Plan

Day	Breakfast	Lunch	Dinner	Dessert
1	Basil Tomato Frittata	Almond Pancakes	Zucchini Salmon Salad	Spinach and Artichoke Dip
2	Coconut Bread	Mouth-watering Pie	Pan Fried Salmon	Buffalo Dip
3	Chia Spinach Pancakes	Peanut Butter and Cacao Breakfast Quinoa	Grilled Salmon with Pineapple Salsa	Potato Wedges
4	Olive Cheese Omelet	Chicken Omelet	Mediterranean Chickpea Salad	Dill Hummus
5	Feta Kale Frittata	Almond Coconut Cereal	Warm Chorizo Chickpea Salad	Latte Pudding
6	Fresh Berry Muffins	WW Salad in a Jar	Tomato Fish Bake	Peanut Butter
7	Cheese Zucchini Eggplant	Almond Porridge	Garlicky Tomato Chicken Casserole	Vegan Crackers
8	Broccoli Nuggets	Special Almond Cereal	Chicken Cacciatore	Spelt Banana Bread
9	Cauliflower Frittata	Bacon and Lemon spiced Muffins	Fennel Wild Rice Risotto	Yeast-Free Spelt Bread
10	Coconut Kale Muffins	Greek Style Mini Burger Pies	Wild Rice Prawn Salad	Flatbread

11	Protein Muffins	Awesome Avocado Muffins	Chicken Broccoli Salad with Avocado Dressing	Chickpea Loaf
12	Healthy Waffles	Raw-Cinnamon-Apple Nut Bowl	Seafood Paella	Zucchini Bread Pancakes
13	Cheese Almond Pancakes	Family Fun Pizza	Herbed Roasted Chicken Breasts	Kamut and Raisin Pancakes
14	Vegetable Quiche	Tasty WW Pancakes	Marinated Chicken Breasts	Spelt and Strawberry Waffles
15	Pumpkin Muffins	Slow Cooker Savory Butternut Squash Oatmeal	Greek Style Quesadillas	Chickpea and Quinoa Burgers
16	Pancakes with Berries	Yummy Smoked Salmon	Creamy Penne	Teff Burgers
17	Omelette À La Margherita	WW Breakfast Cereal	Light Paprika Moussaka	Chickpea Nuggets
18	Porridge with Walnuts	Avocados Stuffed with Salmon	Cucumber Bowl with Spices and Greek Yogurt	Pumpkin Spice Crackers
19	Alkaline Blueberry Spelt Pancakes	Green Lamb Curry	Stuffed Bell Peppers with Quinoa	Spicy Roasted Nuts
20	Ancho Tilapia on Cauliflower Rice	Lemon Lamb Chops	Mediterranean Burrito	Potato Chips

Breakfast Recipes

1. Pancakes with berries

Preparation Time: 5 minutes

Cooking Time: 20 minutes

Servings: 2

Ingredients:

- Pancake:
- 1 egg
- 50 g spelled flour
- 50 g almond flour
- 15 g coconut flour
- 150 ml of water • salt

Filling:

- 40 g mixed berries

- 10 g chocolate
- 5 g powdered sugar
- 4 tbsp yogurt

Directions:

1. Put the flour, egg, and some salt in a blender jar.
2. Add 150 ml of water.
3. Mix everything with a whisk.
4. Mix everything into a batter.
5. Heat a coated pan.
6. Put in half of the batter.
7. Once the pancake is firm, turn it over.
8. Take out the pancake, add the second half of the batter to the pan and repeat.
9. Melt chocolate over a water bath.
10. Let the pancakes cool.
11. Brush the pancakes with the yogurt.

12. Wash the berry and let it drain.

13. Put berries on the yogurt.

14. Roll up the pancakes.

15. Sprinkle them with the powdered sugar.

16. Decorate the whole thing with the melted chocolate.

Nutrition:

kcal: 298

Carbohydrates: 26 g

Protein: 21 g

Fat: 9 g

2. Omelet with tomatoes and spring onions

Preparation Time: 5 minutes

Cooking Time: 20 minutes

Servings:

Ingredients:

- 6 eggs
- 2 tomatoes
- 2 spring onions
- 1 shallot
- 2 tbsp butter
- 1 tbsp olive oil
- 1 pinch of nutmeg
- salt
- pepper

Directions:

1. Whisk the eggs in a bowl.

2. Mix them together and season them with salt and pepper.
3. Peel the shallot and chop it up.
4. Clean the onions and cut them into rings.
5. Wash the tomatoes and cut them into pieces.
6. Heat butter and oil in a pan.
7. Braise half of the shallots in it.
8. Add half the egg mixture.
9. Let everything set over medium heat.
10. Scatter a few tomatoes and onion rings on top.
11. Repeat with the second half of the egg mixture.
12. At the end, spread the grated nutmeg over the whole thing.

Nutrition:

kcal: 263

Carbohydrates: 8 g Protein: 20.3 g

Fat: 24 g

3. Omelet à la Margherita

Preparation Time: 10 minutes

Cooking Time: 20 minutes

Servings: 2

Ingredients:

- 3 eggs
- 50 g parmesan cheese
- 2 tbsp heavy cream
- 1 tbsp olive oil
- 1 teaspoon oregano
- nutmeg
- salt
- pepper
- For covering:
- 3 - 4 stalks of basil
- 1 tomato

- 100 g grated mozzarella

Directions:

1. Mix the cream and eggs in a medium bowl.
2. Add the grated parmesan, nutmeg, oregano, pepper and salt and stir everything.
3. Heat the oil in a pan.
4. Add 1/2 of the egg and cream to the pan.
5. Let the omelet set over medium heat, turn it, and then remove it.
6. Repeat with the second half of the egg mixture.
7. Cut the tomatoes into slices and place them on top of the omelets.
8. Scatter the mozzarella over the tomatoes.
9. Place the omelets on a baking sheet.
10. Cook at 180 degrees for 5 to 10 minutes.

11. Then take the omelets out and decorate them with the basil leaves.

Nutrition:

kcal: 402

Carbohydrates: 7 g

Protein: 21 g

Fat: 34 g

Lunch Recipes

4. Flavorful Taco Soup

Preparation Time: 5 minutes

Cooking Time: 15

Servings: 8

Ingredients:

- 1 lb. of Ground beef
- 3 tablespoons of Taco seasoning, divided
- 4 cup of Beef bone broth
- 2 14.5-oz cans of Diced tomatoes
- 3/4 cup of Ranch dressing

Directions:

1. Put the ground beef into a pot and place over medium high heat and cook until brown, about ten minutes.

2. Add in ¾ cup of broth and two tablespoons of taco seasoning. Cook until part of the liquid has evaporated.

3. Add in the diced tomatoes, rest of the broth, and rest of the taco seasoning. Stir to mix, then simmer for ten minutes.

4. Remove the pot from heat, and add in the ranch dressing. Garnish with cilantro and cheddar cheese. Serve.

Nutrition:

Calories: 309

Fat: 24g

Protein: 13g

5. Delicious Instant Pot Buffalo Chicken Soup

Preparation Time: 10 minutes Cooking Time: 20 minutes

Servings: 6

Ingredients:

- 1 tablespoon of Olive oil • 1/2 Onion, diced)
- 1/2 cup of Celery, diced
- 4 cloves of Garlic, minced
- 1 lb. of Shredded chicken, cooked
- 4 cup of Chicken bone broth, or any chicken broth
- 3 tablespoons of Buffalo sauce
- 6 oz of Cream cheese • 1/2 cup of Half & half

Directions:

1. Switch the instant pot to the sauté function. Add in the chopped onion, oil, and celery. Cook until the onions are brown and translucent, about ten minutes.

2. Add in the garlic and cook until fragrant, about one minute. Switch off the instant pot.

3. Add in the broth, shredded chicken, and buffalo sauce. Cover the instant pot and seal. Switch the soup feature on and set time to five minutes.

4. When cooked, release pressure naturally for five minutes and then quickly.

5. Scoop out one cup of the soup liquid into a blender bowl, then add in the cheese and blend until smooth. Pour the puree into the instant pot, then add in the calf and half and stir to mix.

6. Serve.

Nutrition:

Servings: 1 cup Calories: 270 Protein: 27g

Fat: 16g

Carbohydrates: 4g

6. Creamy Low Carb Cream of Mushroom Soup

Preparation Time: 15 minutes

Cooking Time: 15 minutes

Servings: 5

Ingredients:

- 1 tablespoons of Olive oil
- 1/2 Onion, diced • 20 oz of Mushrooms, sliced
- 6 cloves of Garlic, minced
- 2 cup of Chicken broth • 1 cup of Heavy cream
- 1 cup of Unsweetened almond milk
- 3/4 teaspoon of Sea salt • 1/4 teaspoon of Black pepper

Directions:

1. Place a pot over medium heat and add in olive oil. Add in the mushrooms and onions and cook until browned, about fifteen minutes. Next, add in the garlic and cook for another one minute.

2. Add in the cream, chicken broth, sea salt, almond milk, and black pepper. Cook until boil, then simmer for fifteen minutes.

3. Puree the soup using an immersion blender until smooth. Serve.

Nutrition:

Servings: 1 cup

Calories: 229

Fat: 21g

Protein: 5g

Carbohydrates: 8g

Dinner Recipes

7. Chicken Broccoli Salad with Avocado Dressing

Preparation Time: 5 minutes

Cooking Time: 40 minutes

Servings: 6

Ingredients:

- 2 chicken breasts
- 1 pound broccoli, cut into florets
- 1 avocado, peeled and pitted
- ½ lemon, juiced
- 2 garlic cloves
- ¼ teaspoon chili powder
- ¼ teaspoon cumin powder

- Salt and pepper to taste

Directions:

1. Cook the chicken in a large pot of salty water.

2. Drain and cut the chicken into small cubes. Place in a salad bowl.

3. Add the broccoli and mix well.

4. Combine the avocado, lemon juice, garlic, chili powder, cumin powder, salt and pepper in a blender. Pulse until smooth.

5. Spoon the dressing over the salad and mix well.

6. Serve the salad fresh.

Nutrition:

Calories: 195

Fat: 11g

Protein: 14g

Carbohydrates: 3g

8. Seafood Paella

Preparation Time: 5 minutes

Cooking Time: 40 minutes

Servings: 8

Ingredients:

• 2 tablespoons extra virgin olive oil

• 1 shallot, chopped

• 2 garlic cloves, chopped

• 1 red bell pepper, cored and diced

• 1 carrot, diced

• 2 tomatoes, peeled and diced

• 1 cup wild rice

• 1 cup tomato juice

• 2 cups chicken stock

• 1 chicken breast, cubed

• Salt and pepper to taste

- 2 monkfish fillets, cubed
- ½ pound fresh shrimps, peeled and deveined
- ½ pound prawns
- 1 thyme sprig
- 1 rosemary sprig

Directions:

1. Heat the oil in a skillet and stir in the shallot, garlic, bell pepper, carrot and tomatoes. Cook for a few minutes until softened.
2. Stir in the rice, tomato juice, stock, chicken, salt and pepper and cook on low heat for 20 minutes.
3. Add the rest of the ingredients and cook for 10 additional minutes.
4. Serve the paella warm and fresh.

Nutrition:

Calories: 245 Fat: 8g Protein: 27g

Carbohydrates: 20.6g

9. Herbed Roasted Chicken Breasts

Preparation Time: 5 minutes

Cooking Time: 40 minutes

Servings: 4

Ingredients:

• 2 tablespoons extra virgin olive oil

• 2 tablespoons chopped parsley

• 2 tablespoons chopped cilantro

• 1 teaspoon dried oregano

• 1 teaspoon dried basil

• 2 tablespoons lemon juice

• Salt and pepper to taste

• 4 chicken breasts

Directions:

1. Combine the oil, parsley, cilantro, oregano, basil, lemon juice, salt and pepper in a bowl.

2. Spread this mixture over the chicken and rub it well into the meat.

3. Place in a deep-dish baking pan and cover with aluminum foil.

4. Cook in the preheated oven at 350F for 20 minutes then remove the foil and cook for 20 additional minutes.

5. Serve the chicken warm and fresh with your favorite side dish.

Nutrition:

Calories: 330

Fat: 15g

Protein: 40.7g

Carbohydrates: 1g

Meat Recipes

10. Teriyaki Glazed Halibut Steak

Preparation Time: 30 minutes

Cooking Time: 10-15 minutes

Servings: 3

Ingredients:

- 1-pound halibut steak (1 lean)

For the Marinade:

- 3 oz. soy sauce, low sodium (1/4 condiment)
- ½ cup mirin (1/4 condiment)
- 2 tbsp. lime juice (1/8 condiment)
- ¼ cup sugar (1/8 condiment)
- ¼ cup orange juice (1/8 condiment)
- ¼ tsp. ginger ground (1/8 condiment)

- ¼ tsp. crushed red pepper flakes (1/8 condiment)
- 1 each garlic clove (smashed) (1/8 condiment)

Direction:

1. Place all ingredients for the teriyaki glaze/marinade in a saucepan. Bring to a boil and reduce by half, then allow to cool.
2. When it cools, pour half of the icing/marinade into a zip-up bag along with the halibut, then refrigerate for 30 minutes.
3. Preheat Air fryer to 390 ° F. Place marinated halibut in the Air fryer and cook 10-12 minutes. Rub some of the remaining glaze on the halibut steak.
4. Spread on white rice with basil/mint chutney.

Nutrition:

116 Calories

7g Fat

7.2g Protein

11. Pancetta Chops with Pineapple-Jalapeno Salsa

Preparation Time: 20 minutes

Cooking Time: 20 minutes

Servings: 3

Ingredients:

- 3 pieces of Pancetta Chops (roughly 10 ounces each) (1 lean)
- 2 tablespoons parsley (1/2 green)
- 1 tablespoon of ground Coriander (1/4 condiment)
- ¾ cup of olive oil (1/4 condiment)
- 1 tablespoon of finely chopped rosemary (1/4 green)
- 4 ounces of tomatoes, diced (1/4 green)
- 2 cloves of garlic, chopped (1/4 condiment)
- 4 ounces of pineapple, diced (1/2 healthy fat)
- 8 Jalapenos (1/2 green)
- 3 tsps. of Dijon Mustard (1/4 condiment)

- 1½ tsp. of sugar (1/8 condiment)
- 4 ounces of lemon juice (1/8 condiment)
- 3 tbsp. of finely chopped Cilantro (1/2 green)
- 2½ tsp. of salt (1/8 condiment)

Direction:

1. Place the rosemary, sugar, mustard, and coriander, ¼ cup of olive oil, 1 tablespoon of coriander, 1 ½ teaspoons of salt and 1 tablespoon of parsley in a mixing bowl and mix thoroughly. Add the bacon cutlets and mix.

2. Fill in marinade into a resalable plastic bag and refrigerate for about 3 hours.

3. Heat your deep fryer to 390 ° F.

4. Place the jalapenos in a bowl and season with 1 tsp. of oil to cover them evenly. Transfer the jalapenos to the air fryer and cook for about 7 minutes.

5. Once cooled, peel, remove the seeds and chop the jalapenos into small pieces and transfer them to a bowl. Add the pineapple, tomatoes, garlic and lemon juice, the rest of the oil, parsley, coriander and salt. Stir and set the sauce aside.

6. Remove the bacon chops from the refrigerator and allow to rest for 30 minutes at room temperature before cooking.

7. Put the ribs in the air fryer and roast at 390 ° F for about 12 minutes. The bacon cutlets are well cooked when the internal temperature is 140 ° F.

Nutrition:

104 Calories

8.7g Fat

6.7g Protein

12. Air Fryer Cheesy Pork Chops

Preparation Time: 5 minutes

Cooking Time: 8 minutes

Servings: 2

Ingredients:

- 4 lean pork chops (2 leans)
- Salt: half tsp. (1/4 condiment)
- Garlic powder: ½ tsp. (1/4 condiment)
- Shredded cheese: 4 tbsp. (1 healthy fat)
- Chopped cilantro (1 green)

Direction:

1. Let the air fryer preheat to 350 degrees.
2. With garlic, coriander and salt, rub the pork chops. Put the air fryer on. Let it cook for four minutes. Turn them over and then cook for extra two minutes.

3. Drizzle the cheese on top and cook for another two minutes or until the cheese has melted.

4. Serve with salad.

Nutrition:

467 Calories

61g Protein

22g Fat

13. Bacon and Garlic Pizzas

Preparation Time: 10 minutes

Cooking Time: 10 minutes

Servings: 4

Ingredients:

- 4 dinner rolls, frozen
- 4 garlic cloves minced
- ½ tsp. oregano dried
- ½ tsp. garlic powder
- 1 cup ketchup
- 8 bacon slices, cooked and chopped
- 1 and ¼ cups cheddar cheese, grated

Directions:

1. Put the rolls on a surface and press them to obtain 4 ovals.
2. Spray each oval with cooking spray, transfer them to the air fryer and cook at 370 ° F for 2 minutes.

3. Spread the ketchup on each oval, divide the garlic, sprinkle with oregano and garlic powder and garnish with bacon and cheese.

4. Return the pizzas to your hot air fryer and cook them at 370 ° F for another 8 minutes.

5. Serve hot for lunch.

Nutrition:

104 Calories

9g Fat

8.5g Protein

14. Cornbread with Pulled Pancetta

Preparation Time: 24 minutes

Cooking Time: 19 minutes

Servings: 2

Ingredients:

- 2½ cups pulled Pancetta (1 lean)
- 1 tsp. dried rosemary (1/4 green)
- 1/2 tsp. chili powder (1/4 condiment)
- 3 cloves garlic (1/4 condiment)
- 1/2 recipe cornbread (1 healthy fat)
- 1/2 tablespoon brown sugar (1/4 condiment)
- 1/3 cup scallions, thinly sliced (1/2 green)
- 1 tsp. sea salt (1/8 condiment)

Direction:

1. Preheat a pan over medium heat; now cook the shallots together with the garlic and the pulled bacon.

2. Next, add the sugar, chili powder, rosemary and salt. Cook, stirring regularly until thickened.

3. Preheat your air fryer to 335 ° F. Now, coat two mini loaf pans with cooking spray. Add the pulled bacon mixture and spread over the bottom with a spatula.

4. Spread the previously prepared cornbread batter over the spicy pulled bacon mixture.

5. Bake this cornbread in a preheated air fryer until a centered tester is clean, or for 18 minutes.

Nutrition:

117 Calories

9.4g Fat

11g Protein

15. Apricot-Glazed Pork Chops

Preparation Time: 15 minutes

Cooking Time: 6 minutes

Servings: 6

Ingredients:

- 6 boneless pork chops
- ½ cup of apricot
- 1 tablespoon of balsamic vinegar
- 2 teaspoons of olive oil
- Black pepper to taste

Directions:

1. Add oil to your cooker and heat on "chicken/meat," leaving the lid off.

2. Sprinkle black pepper on the pork chops.

3. Roast chops in the cooker on each side till golden.

4. Mix balsamic and apricot preserving together.

5. Pour over the pork and seal the cooker lid.

6. Adjust cook time to 6 minutes.

7. When the time is up, hit “cancel” and quick-release.

8. Test temperature of pork—it should be 145oF.

9. Allow to rest for 5 minutes before serving!

Nutrition:

Total calories: 296 Protein: 20 g Carbs: 18 g

Fat: 16 g

Fiber: 0

16. Simple Beef Stir-fry

Cooking Time: 30 minutes

Servings: 4

Ingredients:

- 2 cups of vegetable stock 2 tablespoons of soy sauce
- garlic cloves; chopped
- 2 teaspoons of chili powder
- 1 pound of top sirloin beef; thinly sliced
- 3 cups of broccoli; chopped into florets
- 1 cup of cremini mushrooms; sliced
- 1 cup of sugar snaps peas
- green onions; sliced
- 1 tablespoon of fresh ginger; peeled and sliced

- 2 tablespoons of grapeseed oil

Directions:

1. Prepare the marinade in a shallow dish or a zip-lock bag, mix vegetable stock, soy sauce, and chili powder. If you desire more spices, add ½ teaspoon of cayenne pepper. Toss the meat in the sauce and marinate for 10-15 minutes.

2. On high heat, add oil to the wok and when hot, put in ginger, broccoli, mushrooms, peas, green onions, and ¼ of the marinade, cook for about 3 minutes or until the broccoli softens. Add beef and the remaining marinade and cook until beef is browned. Serve hot.

Nutrition:

Calories: 412 Fat: 12 g Carbs: 14 g

Protein: 24 g

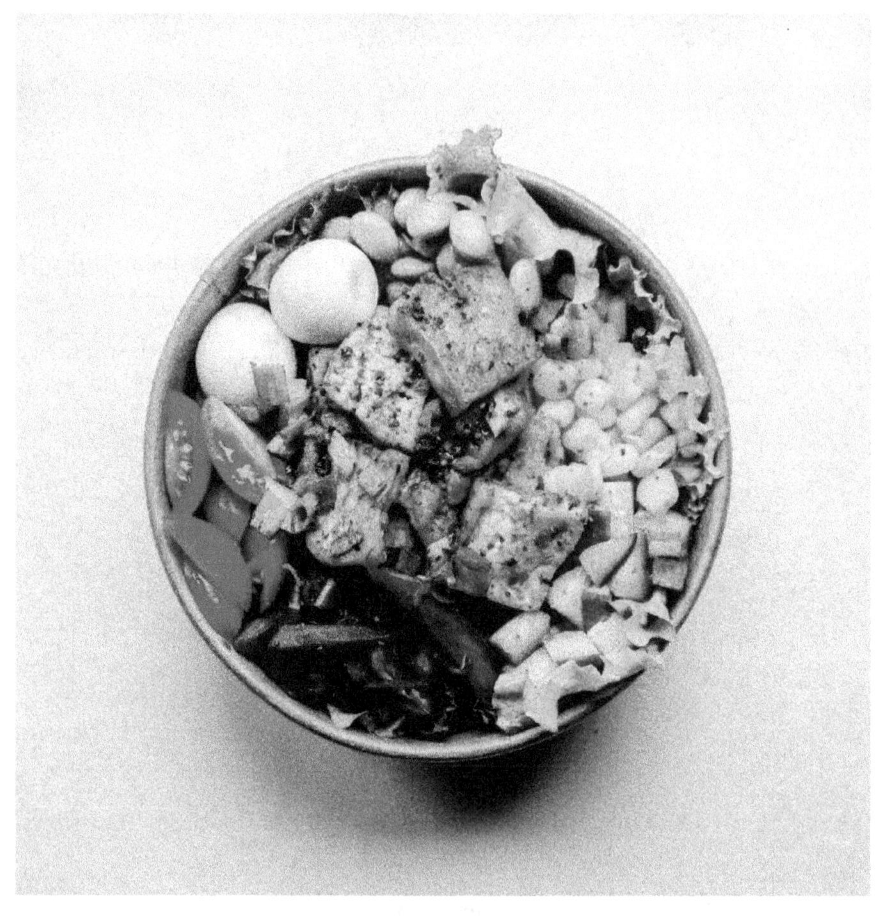

Poultry Recipes

17. Chicken with Avocado Salsa

Preparation Time: 15 minutes.

Cooking Time: 42 minutes.

Serving: 2

Ingredients:

- 1 ½ pounds boneless chicken breasts

Marinade

- 2 garlic cloves, minced
- 3 tablespoons olive oil
- ¼ cup cilantro, chopped
- Juice of 1 lime

- ½ teaspoons salt
- ¼ teaspoons black pepper

Avocado Salsa

- 2 avocados, diced
- 2 small tomato, chopped
- ¼ cup red onion, chopped
- 1 jalapeno, deseeded and chopped
- 1/4 cup cilantro, chopped
- Juice of 1 lime
- Black pepper and salt to taste

Preparation:

1. Mix all the marinade ingredients in a bowl.
2. Pound and flatten each chicken breast into ¼ inch thickness.

3. Add this chicken to the marinade, mix well, cover and refrigerate for 30 minutes.

4. Grill the chicken for 6 minutes per side in a preheated grill.

5. Serve the chicken with the avocado salsa.

6. Mix all the avocado salsa ingredients in a bowl.

7. Enjoy.

Serving Suggestion: Serve the chicken with cauliflower rice.

Variation Tip: Add dried herbs to the mixture for seasoning.

Nutrition Per Serving:

Calories 331

Fat 20g Sodium 941mg Carbs 30g Fiber 0.9g

Sugar 1.4g Protein 24.6g

18. Chicken Piccata

Preparation Time: 15 minutes.

Cooking Time: 10 minutes.

Serving: 8

Ingredients:

- 8 boneless chicken breast halves
- 3 teaspoons olive oil
- 2 tablespoons butter
- 1/2 cup all-purpose flour
- 1/2 cup Parmesan cheese, grated
- 1/2 cup egg
- 1/2 teaspoon salt
- 2 tablespoons 1/4 cup dry white wine

- 1/4 cup parsley minced
- 1/8 teaspoon hot pepper sauce
- 5 tablespoons lemon juice
- 3 garlic cloves, minced

Direction:

1. Pound and flatten each chicken piece.
2. Beat egg with hot pepper sauce, garlic, and 2 tablespoons lemon juice in a bowl.
3. Mix flour with salt, parsley, and Parmesan cheese in a bowl.
4. First coat the chicken with the flour mixture then dip in the egg mixture and coat again with the flour mixture.
5. Place the coated chicken a greased skillet and cook for 5 minutes per side.

6. Mix lemon juice, melted butter and remaining wine in a saucepan and boil.

7. Drizzle this sauce over the chicken.

8. Serve warm.

Serving Suggestion: Serve the chicken with a fresh crouton's salad.

Variation Tip: Add a drizzle of cheese on top.

Nutrition Per Serving:

Calories 300

Fat 2g

Sodium 374mg Carbs 30g Fiber 6g

Sugar 3g

Protein 32g

19. Spinach Mushroom Chick

Preparation Time: 15 minutes.

Cooking Time: 43 minutes.

Serving: 4

Ingredients:

- 6 ounces bag raw spinach leaves
- 2 ounces cream cheese
- 2 garlic cloves, minced
- 8 ounces baby bella mushrooms
- 2 teaspoons garlic powder
- 2 teaspoons salt
- 2 teaspoons ground thyme
- 4 chicken breasts

- 4 mozzarella cheese slices

Direction:

1. At 400 degrees F, preheat your oven.
2. Season chicken with thyme, salt and 1 teaspoon garlic powder.
3. Place this chicken in a casserole dish and bake for 15 minutes in the oven.
4. Sauté garlic in a skillet for 1 minute.
5. Stir in spinach and cook for 10 minutes.
6. Add cream cheese then mix well and remove from the heat.
7. Sauté mushrooms with thyme, salt, and 1 teaspoon garlic powder in a skillet for 7 minutes.
8. Stir in cream cheese mixture and mix well.
9. Spread this mixture on top of the baked chicken.

10. Drizzle cheese on top and bake another 10 minutes.

11. Serve warm.

Serving Suggestion: Serve the chicken with toasted bread slices.

Variation Tip: Add butter sauce on top of the chicken before cooking.

Nutrition Per Serving:

Calories 419

Fat 13g

Sodium 432mg

Carbs 9.1g

Fiber 3g

Sugar 1g

Protein 21g

20. Sesame Chicken

Preparation Time: 15 minutes.

Cooking Time: 20 minutes.

Serving: 2

Ingredients:

- 1 lb. boneless chicken breasts, diced
- 1 large head of broccoli, chopped
- 2 red bell peppers, cut into chunks
- 1 cup snap peas
- Salt and black pepper, to taste
- Sesame seeds and green onions

Sauce:

- 1/4 cup soy sauce

- 1 tablespoon sweet chili sauce
- 2 tablespoons honey
- 2 garlic cloves
- 1 teaspoon fresh ginger

Direction:

1. At 400 degrees F, preheat your oven.
2. Mix all the sauce ingredients in a saucepan and cook until it thickens.
3. Remove the sauce from the heat and allow the sauce to cool.
4. Spread the veggies and chicken in a greased baking sheet.
5. Drizzle sauce over the mixture and mix well.
6. Bake the mixture for 20 minutes in the oven.
7. Garnish with sesame seeds.

8. Serve warm.

Serving Suggestion: Serve the chicken with toasted bread on the side.

Variation Tip: Add some canned corn to the meal.

Nutrition Per Serving:

Calories 334

Fat 16g

Sodium 462mg

Carbs 31g

Fiber 0.4g

Sugar 3g

Protein 25.3g

21. Air Fryer Chicken & Broccoli

Preparation Time: 11 minutes

Cooking Time: 15 minutes

Servings: 4

Ingredients:

- Olive oil: 2 Tablespoons (1/8 condiment)
- Chicken breast: 4 cups, bone and skinless (cut into cubes) (2 lean)
- Low sodium soy sauce: 1 Tbsp. (1/8 condiment)
- Garlic powder: half teaspoon (1/8 condiment)
- Rice vinegar: 2 teaspoons (1/8 condiment)
- Broccoli: 1-2 cups, cut into florets (1 green)
- Hot sauce: 2 teaspoons (1/8 condiment)

- Fresh minced ginger: 1 Tbsp. (1/8 condiment)
- Sesame seed oil: 1 teaspoon (1/8 condiment)
- Salt & black pepper, to taste (1/8 condiment)

Directions:

1. In a bowl, add chicken breast, onion, and broccoli. Combine them well.
2. In another bowl, add ginger, oil, sesame oil, rice vinegar, hot sauce, garlic powder, and soy sauce mix it well. Then add the broccoli, chicken, and onions to marinade.
3. Coat well the chicken with sauces. Set aside in the refrigerator for 15 minutes
4. Place chicken mix in one even layer in air fryer basket and cook for 16-20 minutes, at 380 F. halfway through, toss the basket gently and cook the chicken evenly

5. Add five minutes more, if required.

6. Add salt and pepper if needed.

7. Serve warm with lemon wedges

Nutrition:

191 Calories

7g Fat

25g Protein

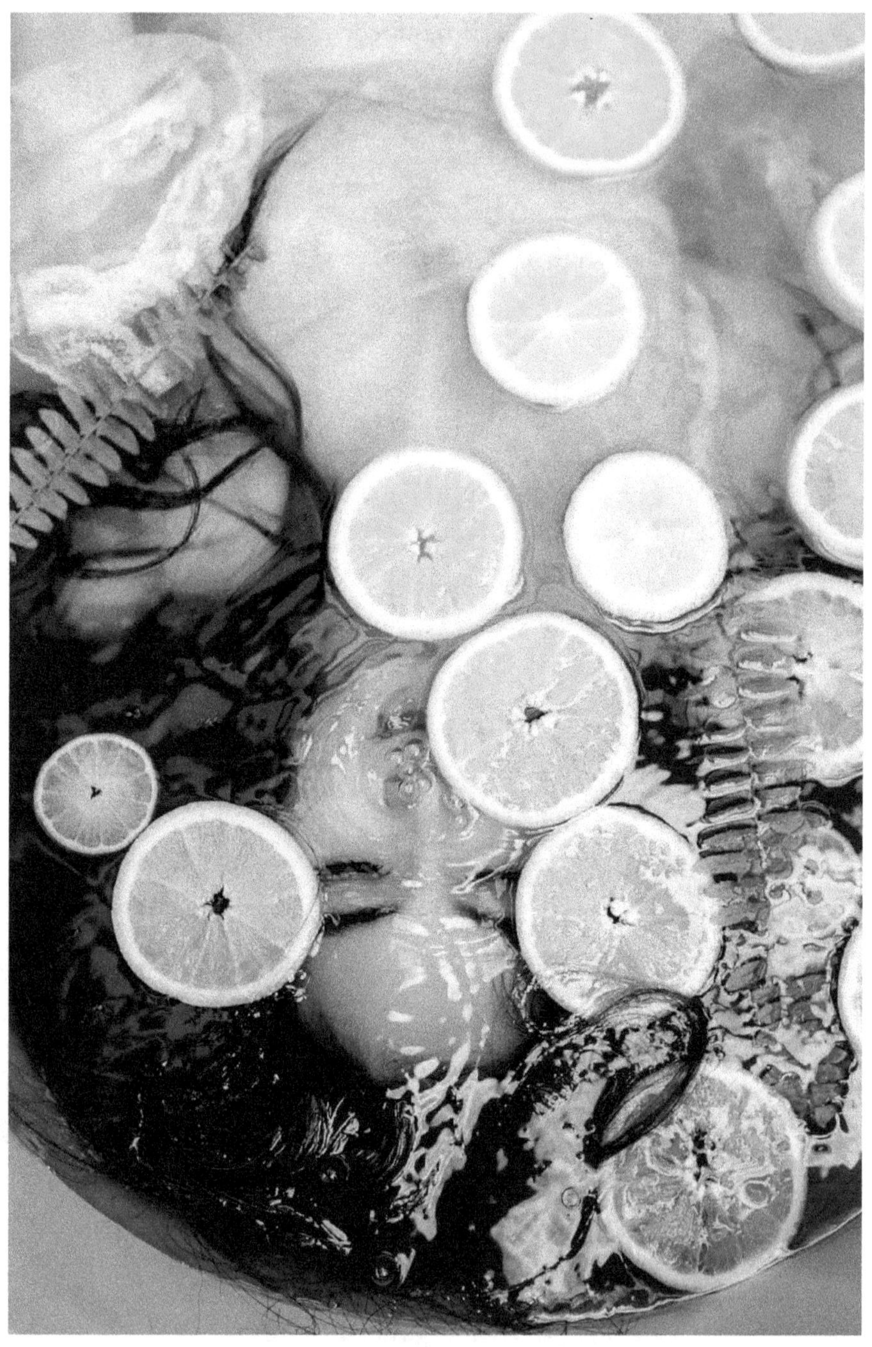

Fish and Seafood Recipes

22. Cilantro Shrimp

Preparation time: 10 minutes

Cooking time: 15 minutes

Servings: 4

Ingredients:

- 1-pound shrimps
- 3 garlic cloves, diced
- ¼ cup fresh cilantro, chopped
- 2 tablespoons butter
- ¼ cup milk
- ½ teaspoon salt

Directions:

1. Put butter in the skillet and bring it to boil.

2. Then add diced garlic and roast it for 3 minutes.

3. Add milk and salt. Bring the liquid to a boil (it will take about 2 minutes).

4. After this, add shrimps and mix up well.

5. Cook the shrimps for 3 minutes over medium heat.

6. Then add fresh cilantro.

7. Close the lid and cook seafood for 5 minutes.

8. Serve the cooked garlic shrimps with cilantro-garlic sauce.

Nutrition: Calories 197, Fat 8g, Fiber 0.1g, Carbs 3.3g, Protein 26.6g

23. Garlicky Clams

Preparation time: 5 minutes

Cooking time: 10 minutes

Servings: 4

Ingredients:

- lbs. clams, clean
- garlic cloves
- ½ cup olive oil
- ½ cup fresh lemon juice
- 1 cup white wine Pepper Salt

Directions:

1. Add oil into the inner pot of the instant pot and set the pot on sauté mode.

2. Add garlic and sauté for 1 minute.

3. Add ride and cook for 2 minutes.

4. Add remaining ingredients and stir well.

5. Seal pot with lid and cook on high for 2 minutes.

6. Once done, allow to release pressure naturally. Remove lid. Serve and enjoy.

Nutrition:

Calorie 332, Fat 13.5g, Carbs 40.5g, Sugar 12.5g, Protein 2.5g, Cholesterol 0 mg

24. Cod Potato Soup

Preparation time: 1 Hour

Cooking time 45 minutes

Servings: 8

Ingredients:

- 2 tablespoons olive oil
- 2 shallots, chopped
- 1 celery stalk, sliced
- 1 carrot, sliced
- 1 red bell pepper, cored and diced
- 2 garlic cloves, chopped
- 1 ½ pounds potatoes, peeled and cubed
- 1 cup diced tomatoes

- 1 bay leaf
- 1 thyme sprigs
- ½ teaspoon dried marjoram
- 2 cups chicken stock
- 6 cups water
- Salt and pepper to taste
- 4 cod fillets, cubed
- 2 tablespoons lemon juice

Directions:

1. Heat the oil in a soup pot and stir in the shallots, celery, carrot, bell pepper, and garlic.
2. Cook for 5 minutes, then stir in the potatoes, tomatoes, bay leaf, thyme, marjoram, stock, and water.

3. Season with salt and pepper and cook on low heat for 20 minutes.

4. Add the cod fillets and lemon juice and continue cooking for 5 additional minutes.

5. Serve the soup warm and fresh.

Nutrition:

Calories 108, Fat 3.9g, Protein 2.2g, Carbs 17g

25. Lemon Swordfish

Preparation time: 6 minutes

Cooking time: 10 minutes

Servings: 2

Ingredients:

- 12 oz swordfish steaks (6 oz every fish steak)
- 1 teaspoon ground cumin
- 1 tablespoon lemon juice
- ¼ teaspoon salt
- 1 teaspoon olive oil

Directions:

1. Sprinkle the fish steaks with ground cumin and salt from each side.

2. Then drizzle the lemon juice over the steaks and massage them gently with the help of the fingertips.

3. Preheat the grill to 395F.

4. Brush every fish steak with olive oil and place it in the drill.

5. Cook the swordfish for 3 minutes from each side.

Nutrition:

Calories 289, Fat 1.5g, Fiber 0.1g, Carbs 0.6g, Protein 43.4g

26. Fish Tacos

Preparation time: 18 minutes

Cooking time: 20 minutes

Servings: 8

Ingredients:

- 4 tilapia fillets
- ¼ Cup fresh cilantro, chopped
- ¼ Cup fresh lime juice
- 2 tbsp paprika • 1 tbsp olive oil
- Pepper • Salt

Directions:

1. Pour 2 cups of water into the instant pot, then place the steamer rack in the pot.

2. Place fish fillets on parchment paper.

3. Season fish fillets with paprika, pepper, and salt and drizzle with oil and lime juice.

4. Fold parchment paper around the fish fillets and place them on a steamer rack in the pot.

5. Once done, release pressure using quick release. Remove lid.

6. Remove fish packet from the pot and open it.

7. Shred the fish with a fork and serve.

Nutrition:

Calories 67, Fat 2.5g, Carbs 1.1g, Sugar 0.2g, Protein 10.8g, Cholesterol 28mg

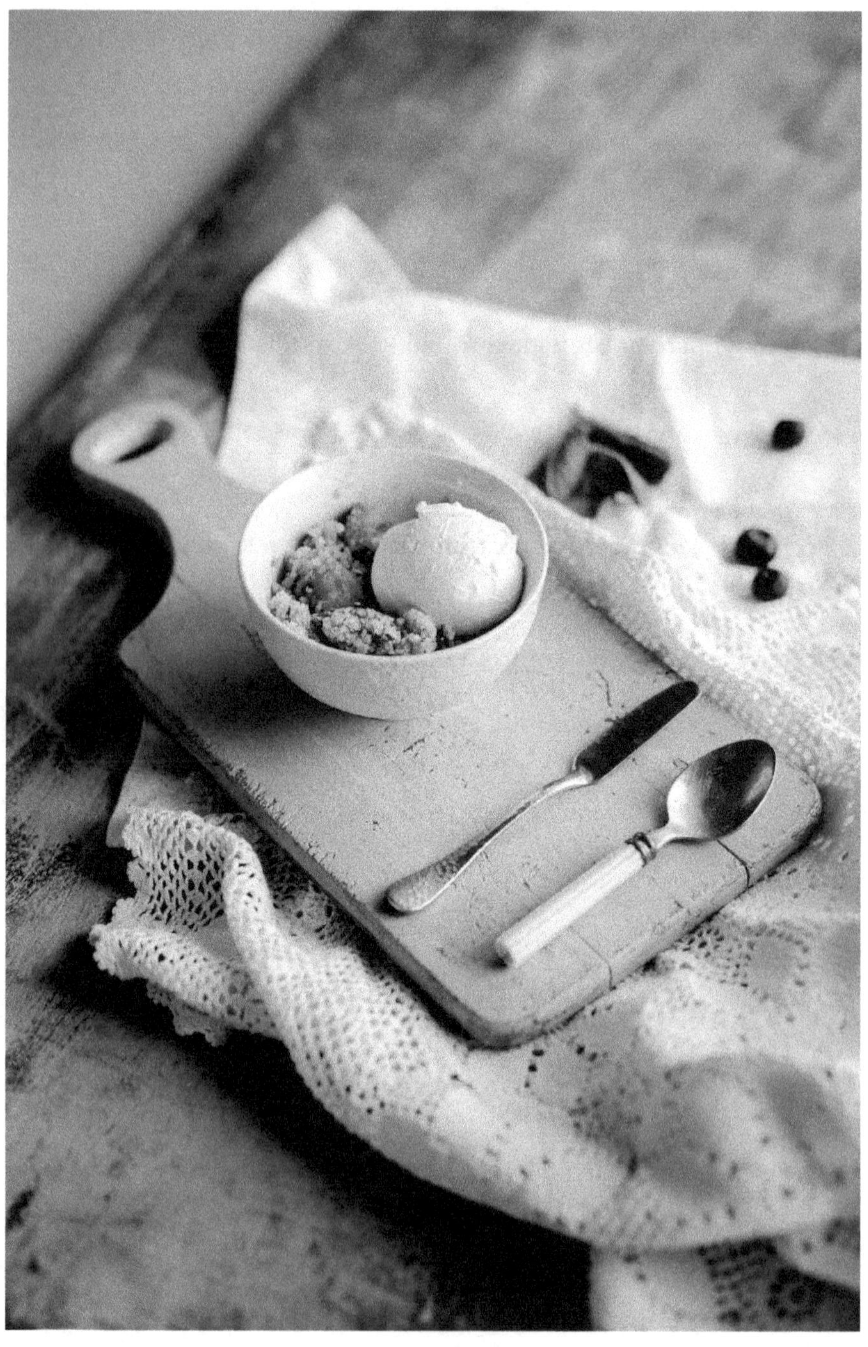

Side Dish Recipes

27. Protein: 5 g Eggplant Tongues

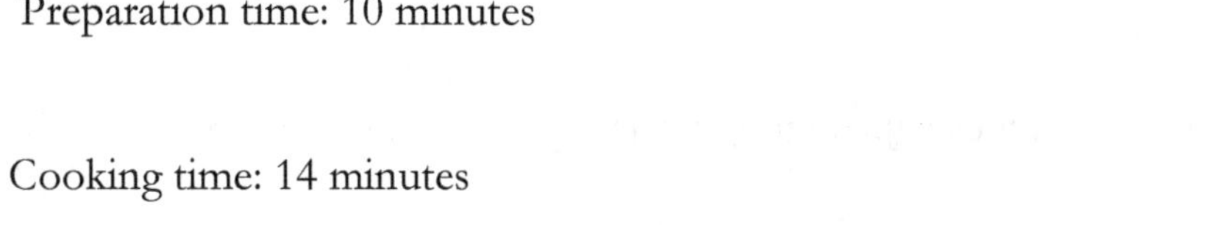

Preparation time: 10 minutes

Cooking time: 14 minutes

Servings: 2

Ingredients:

- eggplants
- 1 teaspoon of minced garlic
- 1 teaspoon of olive oil
- ¼ teaspoon ground black pepper

Directions:

1. Wash the eggplants carefully and slice them.

2. Rub every eggplant slice with the minced garlic, olive oil, and ground black pepper.

3. Place the eggplants in the air fryer basket and cook for 7 minutes from all sides at 375oF.

4. When the eggplant tongues are cooked, serve them immediately!

Nutrition:

Calories: 160

Fat: 3.3 g

Fiber: 19.4 g

Carbs: 32.9 g

28. Protein: 5.5 g Bok Choy and Sprouts

Preparation: 5 minutes Cooking: 20 minutes Servings: 4

Ingredients

- 1 tablespoon of avocado oil
- 1 pound of Brussels sprouts; trimmed and halved
- bok choy head; trimmed and cut into strips
- 1 tablespoon of balsamic vinegar
- A pinch of salt and black pepper
- 1 tablespoon of dill; chopped

Directions:

1 In a pan that fits your air fryer, mix the sprouts with the bok choy and the other ingredients, toss, put the pan in the air fryer and cook at 380oF for 20 minutes.

2 Divide between plates and serve as a side dish.

Nutrition:

Calories: 141

Fat: 3 g

Fiber: 2 g

Carbs: 4 g

Soup and Salad Recipes

29. Flavorful Broccoli Soup

Preparation Time: 10 Minutes

Cooking Time: 4 Hours and 15 minutes

Servings: 6

Ingredients:

- 20 oz. Broccoli florets
- 4 oz. Cream cheese
- 8 oz. Cheddar cheese, shredded
- ½ Tsp. paprika
- ½ Tsp. ground mustard
- 3 Cups chicken stock

- 2 Garlic cloves, chopped
- 1 Onion, diced
- 1 Cup carrots, shredded
- 1/4 Tsp. baking soda
- 1/4 Tsp. salt

Directions:

1. Add all ingredients except cream cheese and cheddar cheese to a crockpot and stir well.
2. Cover and cook on low for 4 hours.
3. Purée the soup using an immersion blender until smooth.
4. Stir in the cream cheese and cheddar cheese.
5. Cover and cook on low for 15 minutes longer.
6. Season with pepper and salt.

7. Serve and enjoy.

Nutrition:

Calories: 275

Fat: 19g

Carbohydrates: 19g

Sugar: 4g

Protein:14g

Cholesterol: 60mg

30. Mexican Chicken Soup

Preparation Time: 10 Minutes

Cooking Time: 4 Hours

Servings: 6

Ingredients:

- 1 ½ lb. Chicken thighs, skinless and boneless
- 14 oz. Chicken stock
- 14 oz. Salsa
- 8 oz. Monterey Jack cheese, shredded

Directions:

1. Place chicken into a crockpot.
2. Pour the remaining ingredients over the chicken.
3. Cover and cook on high for four hours.

4. Remove chicken from the crockpot and shred using forks.

5. Return shredded chicken to the crockpot and stir well.

6. Serve and enjoy.

Nutrition:

Calories: 371

Fat: 15g

Carbohydrates: 7g

Sugar: 2g

Protein: 41g

Cholesterol: 135mg

31. Healthy Chicken Kale Soup

Preparation: 10 minutes Cooking: 6 hours 15 minutes Servings: 6

Ingredients:

- 2 lb. Chicken breasts, skinless and boneless
- 1/4 Cup fresh lemon juice
- 5 oz. Baby kale
- 32 oz. Chicken stock • ½ Cup olive oil
- 1 Large onion, sliced • 14 oz. Chicken broth
- 1 Tbsp. extra-virgin olive oil • Salt

Directions:

1. Heat the extra-virgin olive oil in a pan over medium heat.
2. Season chicken with salt and place in the hot pan.
3. Cover the pan and cook chicken for 15 minutes.

4. Remove the chicken from the pan and shred it using forks.

5. Add shredded chicken to a crockpot.

6. Add sliced onion, olive oil, and broth to a blender and blend until combined.

7. Pour blended mixture into the crockpot.

8. Add remaining ingredients to the crockpot and stir well.

9. Cover and cook on low for 6 hours.

10. Stir well and serve.

Nutrition:

Calories: 493 Fat: 33g Carbohydrates: 8g

Sugar: 9g Protein:47g

Cholesterol: 135mg

32. Creamy Broccoli Cauliflower Soup

Preparation Time: 10 Minutes

Cooking Time: 6 Hours

Servings: 6

Ingredients:

- 2 Cups cauliflower florets, chopped
- 3 Cups broccoli florets, chopped
- 3 ½ Cup's chicken stock
- 1 Large carrot, diced
- ½ Cup shallots, diced
- 2 Garlic cloves, minced
- 1 Cup plain yogurt
- 6 oz. Cheddar cheese, shredded

- 1 Cup coconut milk • Pepper • Salt

Directions:

1. Add all ingredients except milk, cheese, and yogurt to a crockpot and stir well.

2. Cover and cook on low for 6 hours.

3. Purée the soup using an immersion blender until smooth.

4. Add cheese, milk, and yogurt, and blend until smooth and creamy.

5. Season with pepper and salt. 6.Serve and enjoy.

Nutrition:

Calories: 281 Fat: 20g Carbohydrates: 14g Sugar: 9g

Protein: 11g Cholesterol: 32mg

33. Tasty Basil Tomato Soup

Preparation Time: 10 Minutes

Cooking Time: 6 Hours

Servings: 6

Ingredients:

- 28 oz. Can whole peeled tomatoes
- ½ Cup fresh basil leaves
- 4 Cups chicken stock
- 1 Tsp. red pepper flakes
- 3 Garlic cloves, peeled
- 2 Onions, diced
- 3 Carrots, peeled and diced
- 3 Tbsp. olive oil

- 1 Tsp. salt

Directions:

1. Add all ingredients to a crockpot and stir well.

2. Cover and cook on low for 6 hours.

3. Purée the soup until smooth using an immersion blender.

4. Season soup with pepper and salt.

5. Serve and enjoy.

Nutrition:

Calories: 126

Fat: 5g

Carbohydrates: 13g Sugar: 7g

Protein: 5g

Cholesterol: 0mg

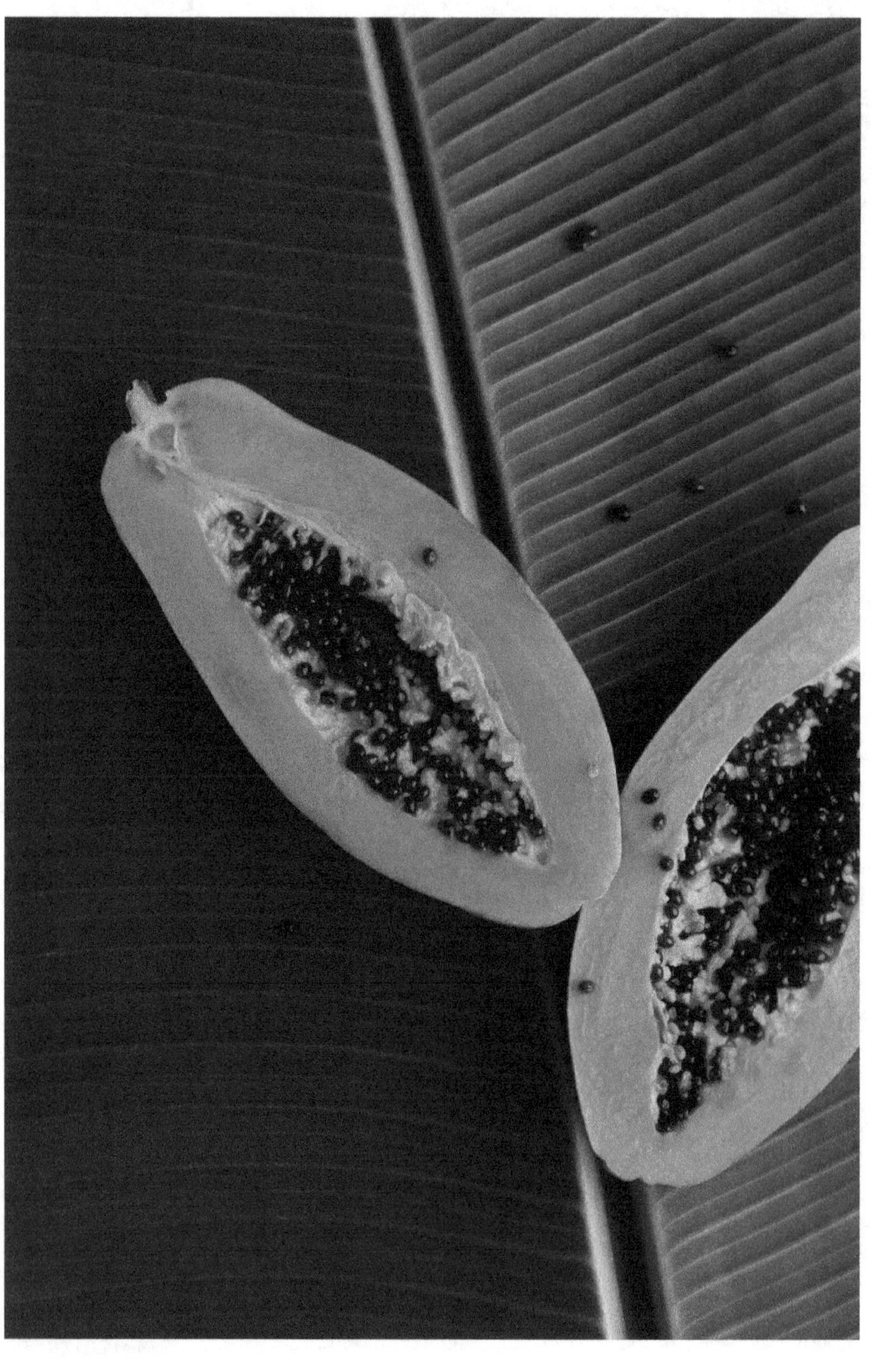

Lean and Green Recipe

34. Chicken Divan

Preparation Time: 15 minutes.

Cooking Time: 41 minutes.

Serves: 8

Ingredients:

- 2 tablespoons olive oil
- 1 lb. boneless chicken breast, diced
- 1 large onion, diced
- 3 garlic cloves, minced
- ¾ teaspoon salt
- ½ teaspoon black pepper

- ½ teaspoon dry thyme
- ¼ cup dry sherry
- 2 cups chicken broth
- ¼ cup all-purpose flour
- 2/3 cup Parmesan cheese, grated
- ¼ cup sour cream
- 2 pieces Broccoli crowns, chopped
- ½ cup water
- 3 tablespoons panko
- ½ teaspoon paprika

Direction:

1. At 400 degrees F, preheat your oven.
2. Grease a 2 ½ quart baking dish with cooking spray.

3. Sauté chicken with 1 tablespoon oil in a skillet until golden brown for 10 minutes.

4. Transfer to a plate, cover with a foil and keep aside.

5. Sauté onion, thyme, black pepper, salt and garlic with 2 teaspoons oil in the same skillet for 4 minutes.

6. Stir in sherry then cook a simmer for 3 minutes.

7. Pour in 1 ½ cup broth then cook on a simmer with occasional stirring.

8. Mix flour with ½ cup broth in a bowl and pour into the skillet.

9. Cook until the mixture thickens then add sour cream and 1/3 cup parmesan.

10. Return the chicken to the mixture and mix well

11. Add broccoli and ½ cup water to a bowl, cover and microwave for 2 minutes.

12. Drain and transfer the broccoli to the chicken then mix well.

13. Spread this chicken mixture in the prepared casserole dish.

14. Drizzle remaining parmesan, panko, paprika and 1 teaspoon oil on top.

15. Bake for 22 minutes in the preheated oven.

16. Serve warm.

Serving Suggestion: Serve the chicken divan with roasted veggies on the side.

Variation Tip: Add peas and corn to the casserole.

Nutritional Information Per Serving:

Calories 334 | Fat 16g |Sodium 462mg | Carbs 31g | Fiber 0.4g | Sugar 3g | Protein 35.3g

35. Spicy Taco Meat

Preparation Time: 15 minutes.

Cooking Time: 16 minutes.

Serves: 6

Ingredients:

- 8 ounces lean ground beef • 8 ounces lean ground turkey breast • ½ cup onion, chopped • 1 (10-ounce) can dice tomatoes
- ½ teaspoon ground cumin
- 1/2 teaspoon ground chipotle chile
- ½ teaspoon dried oregano

Direction:

1. Sauté onion, turkey and beef in a skillet over medium heat for 10 minutes.

2. Transfer the mixture to a plate and keep it aside.

3. Stir in tomatoes, oregano, cumin and chipotle.

4. Sauté for 6 minutes then return the meat mixture.

5. Serve warm.

Serving Suggestion: Serve the taco meat with mashed sweet potato and roasted asparagus on the side.

Variation Tip: Use chicken mince instead of beef.

Nutritional Information Per Serving:

Calories 305 | Fat 25g |Sodium 532mg | Carbs 2.3g | Fiber 0.4g | Sugar 2g | Protein 18.3g

36. Taco Salad

Preparation Time: 15 minutes.

Cooking Time: 10 minutes.

Serves: 6

Ingredients:

- 1 lb. lean ground beef
- 1 tablespoon chili powder
- 8 green onions, chopped,
- 1 head romaine lettuce, chopped
- 1 medium tomato, chopped
- 1 avocado, diced
- 1 4-ounce can olives, sliced
- 1 1/2 cups cheddar cheese, grated

- 1/2 cup plain yogurt
- 1/2 cup salsa

Direction:

1. Sauté beef with black pepper, salt, onions, and chili powder in a skillet until brown.
2. Transfer to a salad bowl then toss in remaining ingredients.
3. Serve.

Serving Suggestion: Serve the salad with toasted bread slices.

Variation Tip: Add crumbled feta cheese on top.

Nutritional Information Per Serving:

Calories 325 | Fat 16g |Sodium 431mg | Carbs 22g | Fiber 1.2g | Sugar 4g | Protein 23g

Vegetables and Sides Recipes

37. Baked Portobello, Pasta, and Cheese

Preparation time: 10 minutes

Cooking time: 30 minutes

Servings: 4

Ingredients:

- 1 cup milk
- 1 cup Mozzarella cheese, shredded
- 1 large garlic clove, minced
- 1 tbsp. vegetable oil
- 1/4 cup margarine
- 1/4 tsp. basil, dried

- 1/4-lb. Portobello mushrooms, thinly sliced
- 2 tbsp. all-purpose flour
- 2 tbsp. soy sauce
- 4 oz. penne pasta, cooked according to manufacturer's directions for cooking
- 5 oz. frozen spinach, thawed, chopped

Directions:

1. Lightly, grease the baking pan of the air fryer with oil. For 2 minutes, heat to 360°F. Add mushrooms and cook for a minute. Transfer to a plate.

2. In the same pan, melt margarine for a minute. Stir in basil, garlic, and flour. Cook for 3 minutes. Stir and cook for another 2 minutes. Stir in half of the milk slowly while whisking continuously. Cook for another

2 minutes. Mix well. Cook for another 2 minutes. Stir in remaining milk and cook for another 3 minutes.

3. Add cheese and mix well.

4. Stir in soy sauce, spinach, mushrooms, and pasta. Mix well. Top with remaining cheese.

5. Cook for 15 minutes at 390°F until tops are lightly browned.

6. Serve and enjoy.

Nutrition:

Calories: 482| Carbs: 32.1 g. | Protein: 16.0 g. | Fat: 32.1 g.

38. Brown Rice, Spinach and Tofu Frittata

Preparation: 20 minutes Cooking: 55 minutes Servings: 4

Ingredients:

- 1/2 cup baby spinach, chopped
- 1/2 cup kale, chopped
- 1/2 onion, chopped
- 1/2 tsp. turmeric
- 1 3/4 cups brown rice, cooked
- 1 flax egg (1 tbsp. flaxseed meal + 3 tbsp. cold water)
- 1 package firm tofu
- 1 tbsp. olive oil
- 1 yellow pepper, chopped
- 2 tbsp. soy sauce

- 2 tsp. arrowroot powder
- 2 tsp. Dijon mustard
- 2/3 cup almond milk
- 3 big mushrooms, chopped
- 3 tbsp. nutritional yeast
- 4 garlic cloves, crushed
- 4 spring onions, chopped
- A handful of basil leaves, chopped

Directions:

1. Preheat the air fryer to 375°F. Grease a pan that will fit inside the air fryer.
2. Prepare the frittata crust by mixing the brown rice and flax egg. Press the rice onto the baking dish until you form a crust. Brush with a little oil and cook for 10 minutes.

3. Meanwhile, heat olive oil in a skillet over medium flame and sauté the garlic and onions for 2 minutes.

4. Add the pepper and mushroom and continue stirring for 3 minutes.

5. Stir in the kale, spinach, spring onions, and basil. Remove from the pan and set aside.

6. In a food processor, pulse together the tofu, mustard, turmeric, soy sauce, nutritional yeast, almond milk, and arrowroot powder. Pour in a mixing bowl and stir in the sautéed vegetables.

7. Pour the vegan frittata mixture over the rice crust and cook in the air fryer for 40 minutes.

Nutrition:

Calories: 226|Carbohydrates: 30.44 g| Protein: 10.69 g. | Fat: 8.05 g

39. Baked Potato Topped with Cream Cheese and Olives

Preparation time: 15 minutes

Cooking time: 40 minutes

Servings: 1

Ingredients:

- 1/4 tsp. onion powder
- 1 medium russet potato, scrubbed and peeled
- 1 tbsp. chives, chopped
- 1 tbsp. Kalamata olives
- 1 tsp. olive oil
- 1/8 tsp. salt
- A dollop of vegan butter

- A dollop of vegan cream cheese

Directions:

1. Place inside the air fryer basket and cook for 40 minutes. Be sure to turn the potatoes once halfway through.

2. Place the potatoes in a mixing bowl and pour in olive oil, onion powder, salt, and vegan butter.

3. Preheat the air fryer to 400°F.

4. Serve the potatoes with vegan cream cheese, Kalamata olives, chives, and other vegan toppings that you want.

Nutrition:

Calories: 504|Carbohydrates: 68.34 g. | Protein: 9.31 g. | Fat: 21.53 g.

40. Banana Pepper Stuffed with Tofu and Spices

Preparation time: 5 minutes

Cooking time: 10 minutes

Servings: 8

Ingredients:

- 1/2 tsp. red chili powder
- 1/2 tsp. turmeric powder
- 1 onion, finely chopped
- 1 package firm tofu, crumbled
- 1 tsp. coriander powder
- tbsp. coconut oil
- 8 banana peppers, top-end sliced and seeded

- Salt to taste

Directions:

1. Preheat the air fryer for 5 minutes.
2. In a mixing bowl, combine the tofu, onion, coconut oil, turmeric powder, red chili powder, coriander powder, and salt. Mix until well-combined.
3. Scoop the tofu mixture into the hollows of the banana peppers.
4. Place the stuffed peppers in the air fryer.
5. Close and cook for 10 minutes at 325°F.

Nutrition:

Calories: 72 |Carbs: 4.1 g. | Protein: 1.2 g. | Fat: 5.6 g.

41. Family Favorite Stuffed Mushrooms

Preparation Time:4 minutes Cooking Time: 12 minutes

Servings: 2

Ingredients:

- 2 teaspoons cumin powder
- 4 garlic cloves, peeled and minced
- 1 small onion, peeled and chopped
- 18 medium-sized white mushrooms
- Fine sea salt and freshly ground black pepper, to your liking
- A pinch ground allspice • 2 tablespoons olive oil

Directions:

1. First, clean the mushrooms; remove the middle stalks from the mushrooms to prepare the "shells".

2. Grab a mixing dish and thoroughly combine the remaining items. Fill the mushrooms with the prepared mixture.

3. Cook the mushrooms at 345 degrees F heat for 12 minutes. Enjoy!

Nutrition:

Calories: 179 | Fat: 14.7g | Carbs: 8.5g | Protein: 5.5g | Sugars: 4.6g | Fiber: 2.6g

42. Cabbage and Radishes Mix

Preparation time: 20 minutes

Cooking time: 15 minutes

Servings: 4

Ingredients:

- 2 cups green cabbage; shredded
- 1/2 cup celery leaves; chopped.
- 1/4 cup green onions; chopped.
- 2 radishes; sliced
- 1 tbsp. olive oil
- 1 tbsp. balsamic vinegar
- 1/2 tsp. hot paprika
- 1 tsp. lemon juice

Directions:

1. In your air fryer's pan, combine all the ingredients and toss well.

2. Place the pan in the fryer and cook at 380°F for 15 minutes.

Divide between plates and serve as a side dish.

Nutrition:

Calories: 130 | Fat: 4 g. | Carbs: 4 g. | Protein: 7 g.

Snacks and Dessert Recipes

43. Chocolate Bars

Preparation Time: 10 minutes

Cooking Time: 20 minutes

Servings: 16

Ingredients:

- 15 oz. cream cheese, softened
- 15 oz. unsweetened dark chocolate
- 1 tsp. vanilla
- 10 drops liquid stevia

Directions:

1. Grease 8-inch square dish and set aside.

2. In a saucepan, dissolve chocolate over low heat.

3. Add stevia and vanilla and stir well.

4. Remove pan from heat and set aside.

5. Add cream cheese into the blender and blend until smooth.

6. Add melted chocolate mixture into the cream cheese and blend until just combined.

7. Transfer mixture into the prepared dish and spread evenly and place in the refrigerator until firm.

8. Slice and serve.

Nutrition:

Calories: 230 Fat: 24 g Carbs: 7.5 g Sugar: 0.1 g Protein: 6 g

Cholesterol: 29 mg

44. Blueberry Muffins

Preparation Time: 15 minutes

Cooking Time: 35 minutes

Servings: 12

Ingredients:

- 2 eggs
- 1/2 cup fresh blueberries
- 1 cup heavy cream
- 2 cups almond flour
- 1/4 tsp. lemon zest
- 1/2 tsp. lemon extract
- 1 tsp. baking powder
- 5 drops stevia

- 1/4 cup butter, melted

Directions:

1. Heat the cooker to 350F. Line muffin tin with cupcake liners and set aside.

2. Add eggs into the bowl and whisk until well mixed.

3. Add remaining ingredients and mix to combine.

4. Pour mixture into the prepared muffin tin and bake for 25 minutes.

5. Serve and enjoy.

Nutrition:

Calories: 190 Fat: 17 g Carbs: 5 g Sugar: 1 g Protein: 5 g

Cholesterol: 55 mg

45. Chia Pudding

Preparation Time: 20 minutes

Cooking Time: 0 minutes

Servings: 2

Ingredients:

- 4 tbsp. chia seeds
- 1 cup unsweetened coconut milk
- 1/2 cup raspberries

Directions:

1. Add raspberry and coconut milk into a blender and blend until smooth.
2. Pour mixture into the glass jar.
3. Add chia seeds in a jar and stir well.

4. Seal the jar with a lid and shake well and place it in the refrigerator for 3 hours.

5. Serve chilled and enjoy.

Nutrition:

Calories: 360

Fat: 33 g

Carbs: 13 g

Sugar: 5 g

Protein: 6 g

Cholesterol: 0 mg

46. Avocado Pudding

Preparation: 20 minutes Cooking: 0 minutes Servings: 8

Ingredients:

- 2 ripe avocados, pitted and cut into pieces
- 1 tbsp. fresh lime juice • 14 oz. can coconut milk
- 2 tsp. liquid stevia • 2 tsp. vanilla

Directions:

1. Inside the blender, add all ingredients and blend until smooth.
2. Serve immediately and enjoy.

Nutrition:

Calories: 317 Fat: 30 g Carbs: 9 g Sugar: 0.5 g Protein: 3 g

Cholesterol: 0 mg

47. Delicious Brownie Bites

Preparation Time: 20 minutes

Cooking Time: 0 minutes

Servings: 13

Ingredients:

- 1/4 cup unsweetened chocolate chips
- 1/4 cup unsweetened cocoa powder
- 1 cup pecans, chopped
- 1/2 cup almond butter • 1/2 tsp. vanilla
- 1/4 cup monk fruit sweetener • 1/8 tsp. salt

Directions:

1. Add pecans, sweetener, vanilla, almond butter, cocoa powder, and salt into the food processor and process until well combined.

2. Transfer brownie mixture into the large bowl. Add chocolate chips and fold well.

3. Make small round shape balls from brownie mixture and place onto a baking tray.

4. Place in the freezer for 20 minutes.

5. Serve and enjoy.

Nutrition:

Calories: 108

Fat: 9 g

Carbs: 4 g

Sugar: 1 g

Protein: 2 g

Cholesterol: 0 mg

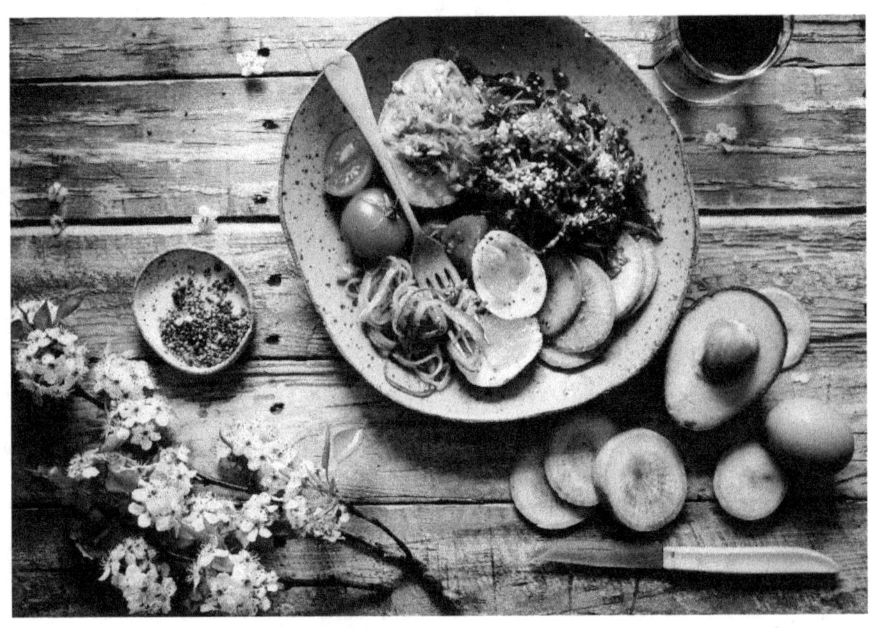

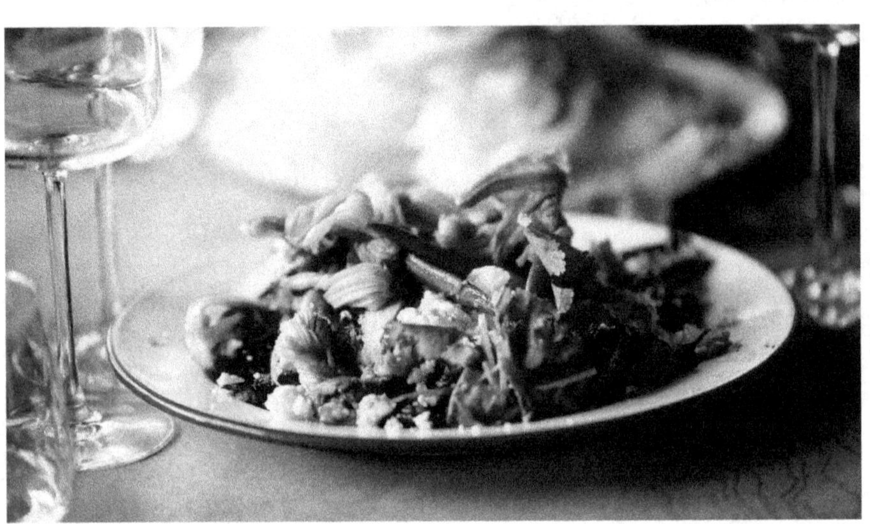

Fueling Recipes

48. Egg and Vanilla Shake

Preparation Time: 5 Minutes Cooking Time: 5 Minutes

Servings: 1

Ingredients:

- 2 sachets Lean & Green Essential Creamy Vanilla Shake
- 16 oz vanilla almond milk, unsweetened
- 2 eggs pasteurized; yolk separated
- ½ tsp rum extract • ¼ tsp nutmeg

Directions:

1. In an air fryer compatible cooking bowl, combine rum extract, vanilla shake, and vanilla almond milk.

2. Place the bowel in the air fryer and warm for 5 minutes at 205°C.

3. Take it out and transfer it into a blender.

4. Add egg yolk and blend until it becomes smoothy.

5. Put the egg white in a small bowl and beat it with a hand blender until it starts to foam.

6. Transfer the beaten egg into a large glass.

7. Pour the vanilla shake mixture over it and sprinkle a pinch of nutmeg.

8. Serve fresh

Nutrition: Calories: 404; Fat: 11g; Protein: 11g; Carbohydrates: 45g

49. Peanut Butter Chocolate Donuts

Preparation Time: 10 Minutes

Cooking Time: 15 Minutes

Servings: 2

Ingredients:

- 3 oz Lean & Green Essential Golden Chocolate Chip Pancakes
- 3 oz Lean & Green Essential Decadent Double Chocolate

Brownie

- 3 tbsp liquid egg substitute
- 1/8 cup vanilla almond unsweetened milk
- ¼ tsp vanilla extract
- ¼ tsp baking powder
- Cooking spray – as required

For glaze:

- ¼ cup peanut butter, ground
- 2 tbs vanilla almond milk, unsweetened

Directions:

1. Preheat the air fryer to 175°C.
2. Place the chocolate pancake chips into a bowl and crumble.
3. Mix it brownies, milk, egg substitute, vanilla extract, and baking powder.
4. Spray some cooking oil onto the donut slots.
5. Transfer the mixture evenly into the 4 slots of the donut pan.
6. Place the pan in the air fryer and bake for 15 minutes until it turns well.
7. After that, take it out from the air fryer and allow it to cool for doing the glazing.

8. For the glazing, combine ground peanut butter and milk in a shallow bowl until it becomes smooth and thin.

9. Dip the donuts into the glaze and decorate with chocolate chips.

Nutrition: Calories: 397; Fat: 15g; Protein: 7g; Carbohydrates: 63g

50. French Toast Sticks

Preparation Time: 5 Minutes

Cooking Time: 4 Minutes

Servings: 2

Ingredients:

- 2 sachets Lean & Green Essential Cinnamon Crunchy O's Cereal
- 2 tbsp cream cheese, low fat, softened
- 6 tbsp liquid egg substitute
- 2 tbsp sugar-free syrup • Cooking spray – as required

Directions:

1. In a blender, blitz Cinnamon Crunchy Os until its consistency turn to look like breadcrumbs.

2. Pour liquid egg substitute and cream cheese into the blender blend until it turns to a dough.

3. Make 6 French toast like sticks out of the dough.

4. Slightly brush the air fryer grill with oil.

5. Place the French toast dough over the grill basket.

6. Set the temperature to 204°C and air fry for 4 minutes.

7. After air frying, serve by topping with sugar-free syrup.

Nutrition: Calories: 92; Fat: 3g; Carbohydrates: 8g; Protein: 7g

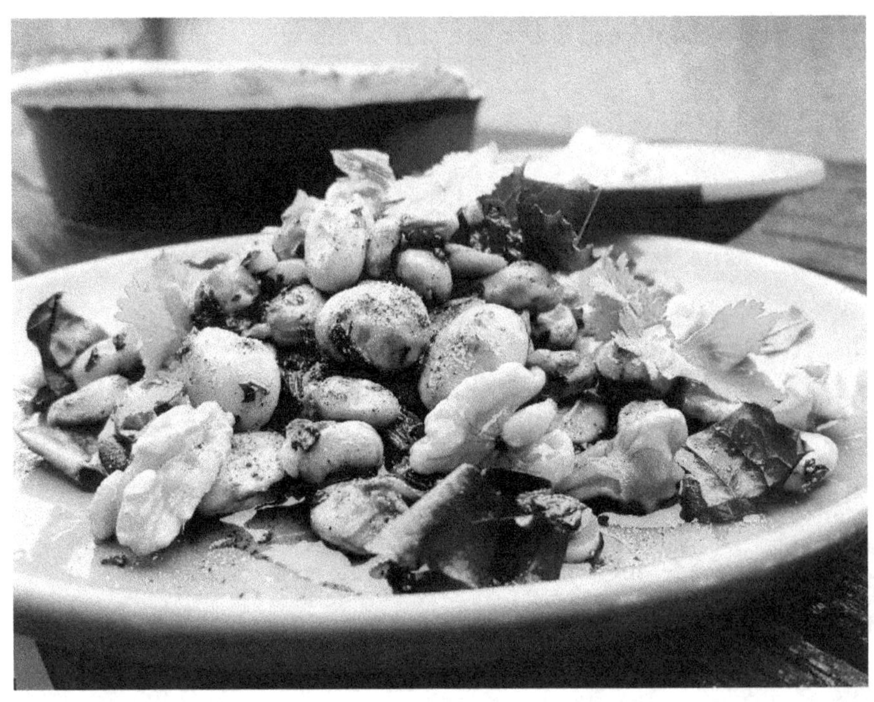

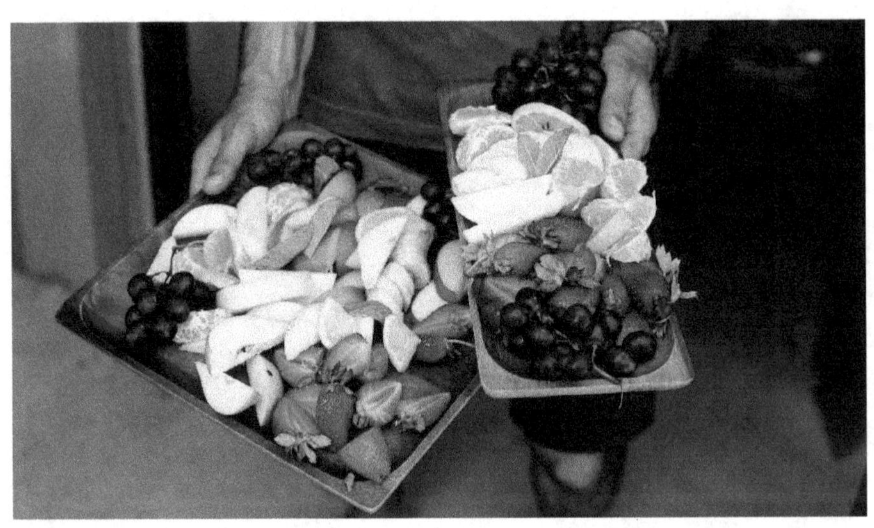

Conclusion

It is the last article in my series on Lean and Green Recipes. Thank you so much for sticking with me all this way, and I hope you found it helpful. I have compiled a series of useful resources at the end of this article, including some wonderful books, websites and podcasts. I can recommend readers who have more knowledge about sustainable living or cooking to interested readers. They helped me a lot over the last few years and I hope they can do the same for you too.

Lean cooking is a style of cooking that emphasizes relatively low-fat content and minimal use of oil. Lean meat, fish, vegetables and grains are cooked in the minimum amount of fat necessary to preserve them. It's not a very customizable way to cook because you can't change the fat content or oil used (you can however swap out all the lean ingredients with higher fat ones).

Green cooking is a style of cooking that emphasizes lessening the environmental impact of your meal preparation by focusing on local, seasonal produce, along with avoiding the use of processed foods or meats that have been produced overseas. As with Lean cooking, it's not very customizable since you're required to buy local and seasonal produce.

The basic idea behind Lean and Green cooking is to approach your weekly meal planning from a perspective of total calories instead of from a perspective of how many calories you are getting from fat or protein. You can use the concepts and recipes I provide to make your own lean meats and green foods, or you can improvise new things.

Because Lean and Green cooking approaches your weekly meal planning from a perspective of total calories instead of from a perspective of how many calories you are getting from fat or protein, it helps you develop a more mindful relationship with food. It's easier to overeat and to consume more calories than you need when you don't pay attention to the actual numbers of food that you're eating. Lean and Green cooking helps break this cycle and make you more aware of your relationship with food in a positive way.

It's also a very simple way to eat, once you figure out what combination of foods works best for your body. And this is where I've found the most appeal for myself personally. My body feels great when I eat a nutritious diet, but I'm also very aware of how many calories I'm eating, and simultaneously, how much fat or protein is in those calories. And if my stomach feels like it's about to boom (which it does sometimes!), I know that there's enough food in my meal that makes me satisfied and not too full.

I hope you can take some of my lessons into your own kitchen. And if you substitute a few ingredients or otherwise make adjustments to suit your tastes, feel free! After all, that's really what creating food is all about: using whatever ingredients you have for what dish you want to create. What matters is the love and care that go into it.

CPSIA information can be obtained
at www.ICGtesting.com
Printed in the USA
BVHW092259210621
610124BV00009B/1635